ESTABLISH TRUST THROUGH
TOUCH WITH MASSAGE

T.R.I.B.E

TOUCH REQUIRES INTEGRITY AND BOLDNESS EFFORTLESSLY

DR. DOMINIQUE M. CARSON, LMP, MMP, H.C

ISBN: 978-1-968061-66-1

Table of Contents

Introduction
by Denise Rivera, LMT

T ake a deep breath… and let it go. You've entered a space created to soothe your senses, spark your creativity, and remind you of something essential — healing begins with presence, and often, with a simple touch.

The T.R.I.B.E book is the beautiful vision of Dr. Dominique Carson, a fellow massage therapist and someone I'm grateful to call a kindred spirit. When she asked me to write this introduction, I was honored — not only because of our shared journey, but because I believe deeply in the message behind these pages. We met while studying massage therapy at Queensborough Community College. We quickly bonded over our shared passion for both communication and healing — she with her journalistic creativity, and I with a background in television production. It became clear early on that we were both drawn to the profound ways the body speaks, holds, and releases — and how powerful it is to listen, both through hands and heart.

Massage is one of the oldest and most universal forms of care. Long before words, there was touch — our hands, the original healing tools, offering comfort, relief, and connection. In today's fast-paced world, massage remains a vital form of self-care — a chance to turn inward, to feel, and to honor the needs of the body. Our bodies are our temples, and all bodies, from all walks of life, deserve the support of healing touch.

This book is a celebration of the wisdom behind touch. Dr. Dominique has transformed the essence of massage — its calm, its connection, its artistry

— into visual form, which has also been introduced in the second version of T.R.I.B.E, written. Each page invites you to slow down, to think about massage with intention, and to reconnect with yourself in a gentle, meaningful way with integrative touchwork. Whether you're a massage therapist, a student of healing arts, or someone simply seeking a moment of peace, we hope this book brings you the same sense of grounding and joy that inspired its creation. So find your favorite spot, grab this compelling book, and let the healing begin.

With gratitude and love, Denise Rivera, LMT

Bio: Denise Rivera is a <u>Licensed Massage Therapist (LMT)</u> with a multifaceted background in therapeutic bodywork and wellness education. She currently practices at ProClinix Sports Physical Therapy & Chiropractic in New York, where she specializes in correcting postural deviations through customized massage techniques. Her modalities include therapeutic massage, deep tissue, Swedish, trigger point therapy, prenatal massage, cupping therapy, manual lymphatic drainage, and myofascial stretching.

In addition to her massage therapy credentials, Denise is a 200-hour Experienced Registered Yoga Teacher (ERYT) with over 15 years of experience. She integrates her yoga expertise into her practice by educating clients on self-care and body awareness, aiming to help them achieve a relaxed, pain-free lifestyle. Denise's commitment to wellness and client-centered care makes her a valuable asset to the healing arts and a trusted practitioner in the field of massage therapy.

Prologue

Legendary Sports Massage Therapist Benny Vaughn said a fantastic quote at the Black Massage Therapist Conference in fall 2024. His exact words were, "touch keeps us connected with our humanness," which describes a profound role of physical connection in our overall well-being, especially for the healing arts profession. After Mr. Vaughn said those words, I started thinking about how touch and massage therapy give clients a sense of comfort and safety through our hands and emotional intelligence, which is crucial for establishing relationships with them. As massage providers, our profession reminds people that touch is an innate desire and need for physical connection and human interaction. It is essential for healing and growth. Touch stimulates the release of oxytocin, the "bonding hormone," which enhances feelings of trust, relaxation, and emotional security. It can also lower stress hormones, improve circulation, and promote mental clarity.

Massage therapy is known for relieving physical tension and reinforcing the body-mind connection with emotional resilience. As massage practitioners, we can assist clients in reconnecting with their bodies and emotions because wellness begins with the hands. Vaughn's philosophy is that healing balances physical, emotional, and psychological health and that touch is more than just a physical act—it is a vital bridge to our shared human experience.

Are you ready to elevate your skill set by mastering the integrity, boldness, awareness, and grace required in the art of touch? Let's begin this journey together.

CHAPTER 1

The Power of Intentional Touch

T ouch is an essential way that we communicate, heal, connect, and celebrate with people, and our hands are a tool to make others feel at ease. Our hands are conduits of energy, support, intention, and care; therefore, we must approach massage therapy purposefully and align our actions with sincere intentions. We transform our touch into a deeply therapeutic experience in the treatment room with 60-, 75-, 90-minute, or 2-hour massages. When we're intentional with our touch and aura, we create healing through every movement and technique because we are aware and present. When practiced with integrity, massage therapy fosters trust, relaxation, tranquility, and profound physical and emotional benefits. In this chapter, we will explore how intentional touch can elevate your skill set and the well-being of your clients.

We must think about the science of touch and how it affects the body and mind. Through countless scientific studies, there are powerful effects of touch through research in neuroscience and psychology. Intentional touch can reduce cortisol levels (the stress hormone), promoting relaxation, increase oxytocin (the "bonding hormone"), fostering feelings of safety and connection, improve circulation, aiding in the delivery of oxygen and nutrients throughout the body, lower blood pressure and heart rate, reducing stress-related symptoms, and alleviate symptoms of anxiety, depression, and PTSD through gentle, therapeutic contact.

Massage therapy is not just about working on muscles; it is about engaging the nervous system, releasing stored trauma, and creating a space where the body feels safe to heal. To practice intentional touch, a massage therapist must be mindful of key elements, such as presence and awareness, pressure and pace, empathy and emotional sensitivity, breathing patterns, and energy. Massage providers must be present to sense the client's need in addition to verbal communication. When the touch feels rushed or fast-paced, it becomes impersonal; a focused touch conveys care and dedication. Once the client feels comfortable with your touch, you can adjust the pressure and pace by paying attention to the depth and rhythm of touch based on their feedback, ensuring effectiveness during the session. When your touch aligns with the client due to your energy and presence before the session, it will allow the client to breathe more comfortably during the session. Encouraging your client to perform deep breathing will amplify the benefits of massage by releasing tension and inhaling relaxation effectively.

As health providers, we must add empathy and emotional sensitivity to the session by realizing that each client has a physical and emotional background. This motivates us to provide compassionate and efficient care and establish a safe space for clients to relax and rejuvenate, building trust. But to enhance intentional touch with clients, massage practitioners must ground ourselves before practice, such as prayer and meditation, to center the energy and omit any negativity before treatment once you're aligned, be mindful with your hand placement before each session, have a moment of stillness by placing your hands gently on the client to introduce yourself before applying pressure on their body. It will also show that the strokes are not rushed and serve a purpose while maintaining your rhythm. As time goes on, check in with the client about pressure and comfort while still observing their body language on the table.

Each client is not a one-size-fits-all, so we must think about the emotional impact of intentional touch, especially for those who are dealing with stress and trauma before or after the treatment room. As massage practitioners, emotional intelligence is crucial to help individuals reconnect with their bodies, especially if they have experienced dissociation, and foster trust in people who may have anxiety around physical contact. Your ability to use touch with empathy and integrity determines how safe and supported a client feels during a session. Every massage session is an opportunity to restore balance, peace, confidence, and relaxation in the client's life.

Licensed Massage Therapist and Educator, Shanese Armstrong, has been in the industry for over a decade, demonstrating a deep dedication to her profession. Armstrong, a proud graduate of the Georgia Massage School in Swannee, GA, was inspired to embark on a massage career after working through her chronic conditions. She was born with hip dysplasia and suffered greatly from back pain and hip pain as a child and into a young adult. Therefore, she felt a strong calling to serve people recovering from an injury or living with a chronic soft tissue condition. She said, "I wanted them to know what it feels like to get relief from their constant pain, to sleep a whole night without awakening from their burning, throbbing pain, and to be truly supported and adequately informed of tools, self-care techniques, and massage treatment options."

Testimonials from Previous and Current Clients: The Difference Intentional Touch Makes

Here are real-life examples of how intentional touch has transformed clients' experiences:

- I had a great experience with Dominique and Daniela. I went for a couples massage, and they were super welcoming and kind. They made us feel comfortable and took the time to get to know us. Our massage was relaxing, and the aromatherapy was the finishing touch. They were accommodating to our individual needs. —K.D. (added their initials for privacy).

- Dominique was amazing! Will be going back just for her. She was attentive and gave me a plan to fix my shoulder issues. —Alexia

- I've been coming to Dominique for years, and they never disappoint! I see her and look forward to each visit. Having a consistent therapist who works with me on issues is so helpful. It's a luxe experience at reasonable prices; I'm so grateful for this spa. —A.S.

- I had a 90-minute hot stone massage. Dominique was very knowledgeable and did a great job. She didn't rush, she paid attention to my problem areas, and I feel very relaxed. I will return for another massage. —Amanda

These testimonials highlight how approaching massage therapy with integrity and boldness can create profound healing experiences for clients. Your hands can heal, comfort, and restore as a massage practitioner. However, practicing intentional touch requires integrity by having ethical standards and prioritizing the well-being of your clients. You must be bold and not shy away from your confidence to provide care and create a safe space for clients. It will be effortless if you're passionate about healing arts because you're developing a practice where healing flows naturally through skillful and mindful touch. When the touch is intentional, your routines and strokes will evolve from robotic to transformative healing.

CHAPTER 2

Integrity in the Healing Arts Field

A s Tension Tamers, we recognize that integrity is the foundation of our massage practice, her technical skills, and years of study. When clients view us, they want to see honesty, professionalism, eagerness, and commitment to our field, and that's why it needs to be embodied in our work. Therefore, there are several principles that we must consider in the healing arts: honesty, confidentiality, professionalism, accountability, compassion, and connection. Being transparent with clients about treatment, skill set, expectations, and limitations is essential. We also have to respect clients' privacy and safeguard their personal information by exceeding standards of conduct such as reliability, punctuality, respect, and hard work. The client will respect us more when we consider our actions and decisions inside and outside the treatment room. Lastly, massage providers will merge compassion and connection to prioritize the clients' well-being with empathy, concern, care, and jovial presence. When these principles are established, they will create a safe and therapeutic environment for prospective and current clients.

We know integrity is crucial in massage and its principles, but why does it matter? Healing arts practitioners' profession is delicate and vulnerable. Without integrity, it can lead to erosion of trust between the practitioner and client since the client's safety is compromised, and ethical violations can result in legal or professional consequences. Subsequently, there are ethical guidelines for massage providers such as "primum non nocere" ("first, do no harm" in Latin), informed consent, client respect, and establishing boundaries in professional relationships. When a practitioner has verbal or written permission from the client, they can explain the nature of the massage modality, possible outcomes from frequent massages, potential risks, and contraindications. We can present our ongoing education and new skills with our verbiage by staying informed about research, techniques, popular modalities, and ethical guidelines. As a result, with the client's consent, we encourage them to make decisions and take charge of their health. We can establish boundaries and professional relationships by avoiding conflicts of interest and inappropriate behavior by having authentic and practical client-practitioner boundaries. When boundaries are in place, we can refrain from exploitation, such as financial and emotional manipulation.

Challenges to Maintaining Integrity

Practitioners may face challenges that test their integrity, such as:

- **Financial Pressures:** The temptation to recommend unnecessary treatments for profit.
- **Client Expectations:** Pressure to promise unrealistic results to maintain clientele.
- **Personal Biases:** Allowing personal beliefs to interfere with professional objectivity.
- **Burnout:** Compassion fatigue leading to decreased ethical vigilance.

Overcoming these challenges requires self-awareness, mentorship, and commitment to professional ethics.

Practical Strategies for Upholding Integrity

To maintain integrity in the healing arts, practitioners can adopt the following practices:

- **Develop Clear Policies:** Having written guidelines on ethical conduct, client confidentiality, and informed consent.
- **Engage in Self-Reflection:** Regularly assessing interactions with clients.
- **Seek Peer Support and Mentorship:** Consulting with colleagues or mentors when faced with ethical dilemmas.
- **Prioritize Self-Care:** Preventing burnout by maintaining a healthy work-life balance and engaging in personal wellness practices.
- **Remain Transparent:** Being honest about treatment limitations and referring clients to other professionals when necessary.

Integrity is not a one-time decision but an ongoing commitment. Healing arts practitioners who embody integrity build lasting, trusting relationships with clients, enhance their field's credibility and professionalism, and have a fulfilling practice rooted in ethical care. By embracing integrity in all aspects of their work, healing professionals contribute to a world where trust, respect, and genuine healing flourish. In the next chapter, we will explore how boldness and confidence contribute to creating a successful and impactful healing practice.

CHAPTER 3

The Language of Touch

In society, touch is recognized as a universal language, and along with words, you can initiate communication, care, community, safety, and connection. In the healing arts, touch is a profound language that speaks directly to the body, mind, and spirit. A skilled practitioner understands that each touch carries meaning, conveying reassurance, healing, and intention without the need for verbal expression.

Touch can soothe anxiety, alleviate pain, and create a sense of security. The way a practitioner applies pressure, adjusts their technique, and maintains presence can determine whether a client feels nurtured, vulnerable, or disconnected. Massage therapists must explore the nuances of the language of touch and how to harness its power for healing. Touch plays an essential role in human development and well-being.

Studies show that intentional touch can release oxytocin, the "bonding hormone," promoting feelings of trust and relaxation, decreasing anger, stress, anxiety, and depression, improving circulation and lymphatic drainage, facilitating physical healing, enhancing proprioception, the body's awareness of itself in space, improving balance and mobility, activating the parasympathetic nervous system, shifting the body into a state of deep relaxation and recovery. The benefits indicate the biological impact of touch, which allows practitioners to use it more effectively in their work.

Yetta Delgado LMBT: MMP, CLT, MLD-C is the founder/Owner of Divine Essence Total Bodycare and a massage continuing education provider. Her massage journey and interaction with human touch began when she was searching for another career field and decided to try Southeastern for Medical Billing and Coding. Her liaison at the time, Kim, asked if she wanted to pursue a career in massage therapy. At first, Delgado didn't have any intention of rubbing up against anyone, and vice versa. But her outlook changed when she received her first massage and stated it made her toes dance, but at the same time, she realized she had neglected her body.

After graduating from massage school, Delgado opened a private practice and now specializes in Lymphedema Recovery Care. She said starting was a rollercoaster ride because she needed to establish boundaries with her clients and knew her time was more valuable. She said people would forget about their appointments or not show up, so she started accepting credit card payments for a no-show fee, making it non-refundable, regardless of the Groupon. The policies motivated Delgado to create office policies and procedures. She genuinely believes that clients and her patients trust her skill set and that she puts in 100% effort during their visit. She continually enhances her education in massage therapy to deepen her knowledge, which she can then pass on to clients, ultimately leading to a more effective recovery path.

There are different forms of touch in healing because not all touch is the same. The touch is different due to quality, intention, and technique, and your touch influences clients when you're following the key forms in healing arts:

1. Grounding Touch:
- A steady, intentional hand placement that reassures and calms.

- Used to establish presence and connection before beginning a session.

2. Energizing Touch:
- Light, rhythmic movements that stimulate circulation and awaken the senses.
- Often used in techniques like lymphatic massage.

3. Releasing Touch:
- Deep, slow pressure that encourages muscle and emotional tension to dissolve.
- Found in deep tissue massage and myofascial release.

4. Nurturing Touch:
- Gentle, flowing movements that provide comfort and emotional security.
- Common in Swedish massage, Reiki, and craniosacral therapy.

5. Listening Touch:
- A touch that "listens" to the body's responses, adjusting accordingly.
- Essential for trauma-informed bodywork and intuitive healing.

6. Intentional Touch:
- Touch with purpose equals transformation
- Mindful of your energy
- Infusing meaning with your touch
- Your touch ensures safety, trust, healing, empowerment, balance, and compassion.

Before each session, take a moment to center yourself, clear distractions, and set an intention for how you wish to support your client. This mindfulness elevates your practice from routine to deeply impactful. Remember, physical touch is interpreted differently across cultures and personal experiences and may be perceived as a form of connection or reserved. Some clients may have a history of trauma, making them more sensitive to certain types of touch. Therefore, make sure you have the 2 C's: consent and communication. The massage practitioner must always ensure the client feels comfortable and in control by explaining techniques beforehand and checking in during the session. When you understand these nuances, practitioners create a safe, inclusive, and respectful healing environment.

Moreover, touch can be revealed through non-verbal cues, so you must take heed to how your client responds on the table. You can review the muscle tension by indicating discomfort, stress, hesitation, or areas that need attention. Another example is shallow breathing because it may signal anxiety, while deep breathing suggests relaxation. Lastly, facial expressions such as a furrowed brow or clenched jaw can indicate tension. A client may be silent on the table, but being attuned to clients' non-verbal cues allows practitioners to adjust their approach and enhance the healing experience.

Stress Slayers can master the art of touch by cultivating presence and awareness, understanding the physiological and emotional effects of different types of touch, respecting personal and cultural sensitivities, and continuously refining their skills through education and experience.

Touch is a silent yet powerful form of communication, and when it's applied with care and intention, it leads to profound healing. When used with integrity, boldness, and care, it becomes one of the most profound tools for healing and human connection. In the next chapter, we will explore how to build trust and establish strong client relationships through ethical touch practices.

CHAPTER 4

Establishing a Fearless Connection: Boldness in Touch

Touch can be an act of courage and confidence. In a world where human interaction is often guarded, the ability to offer intentional, confident, and fearless touch is both rare and powerful. As a healing arts practitioner, being bold in your touch doesn't mean applying pressure without sensitivity—it means standing fully in your presence, confident in your ability to create a safe and transformative experience. Boldness in touch is about clarity, conviction, and connection. Courageous and intentional touch breaks down emotional walls, builds trust, and supports more profound healing. Fearless connection is not reckless—it's mindful, confident, aware, and rooted in integrity.

Boldness in touch is not about force—it's about presence. It means touching with clear intention and unwavering confidence, trusting your training and intuition to guide your hands, creating a brave space where clients feel safe enough to let go, and meeting clients where they are, without hesitation or fear. Practitioners who embrace boldness communicate strength and stability, which are essential for clients navigating physical pain, emotional trauma, or disconnection from their bodies.

Boldness matters in healing because it requires clients to become vulnerable. A practitioner's hesitance or self-doubt can unintentionally communicate uncertainty, which may limit the depth of healing that occurs. A bold and confident touch reassures the client that they are in capable hands, encourages the release of tension and emotional resistance, and helps the body feel secure enough to shift from survival mode to healing mode. When boldness is paired with compassion, it becomes a powerful force for transformation. Boldness thrives within clear, respectful boundaries. Clients are more likely to relax when the practitioner is in control of the session with clarity and purpose, their comfort and consent are prioritized at all times, and the practitioner can handle intense emotional or physical reactions without fear or avoidance. Respectful boldness creates safety. It is not about pushing limits, but expanding what is possible in the healing relationship. Becoming bold in massage therapy takes time, experience, and self-awareness. You can cultivate fearless touch and develop boldness as a practitioner by deepening your education. You must stay curious and learn new modalities and techniques to expand your toolkit. Confidence grows when your knowledge is deep and diverse. Next, ground yourself before every session. The more present you are, the more secure your client will feel. It is time to omit self-doubt by trusting in your hands and your intention. Doubt creates energetic barriers and reflects on positive outcomes and feedback to reinforce your confidence. Your hands often know more than your mind. Embrace your intuition and tune into the subtle messages of the body. Lastly, accept imperfection because you do not have to be perfect to be impactful. Boldness includes the willingness to learn, adjust, grow, and revamp.

However, boldness is never about overpowering the client. It's about reading their cues—verbal and nonverbal, being willing to lead when they're uncertain, and holding steady space when they're releasing or expressing emotion. Sometimes, the boldest thing you can do is to stay with a client in silence, with an open heart and steady hands. Practitioners may hold back their bold touch because of fears of: making a mistake, triggering a client's trauma response, being perceived as inappropriate, and fear of their emotional responses. Therefore, you must address fears that require inner work outside of the treatment room; otherwise, you will find excuses and reasons. As a licensed massage therapist, you can seek out supervision, mentorship, and peer support to normalize these challenges. You can also enroll in trauma-informed training that helps practitioners understand triggers and how to navigate them with care. Lastly, personal therapy or bodywork can support emotional regulation and self-awareness. When the inner issues are addressed, your touch will be fearless. Boldness here means trusting your technique and not shying away from working through tough layers of muscle with care. Boldness involves trusting your intuition and being fully present with your energy field. Even in subtle touch, boldness means confident stillness and deep listening. Boldness may come in the form of leading clients through movement confidently and fluidly. The form of boldness changes with each approach, but the essence remains: presence, clarity, and compassionate leadership.

Fearless connection isn't loud or aggressive. It's steady, open, jovial, and sincere. When practitioners touch with boldness, they show up as leaders in the healing journey, offer clients the safety to be vulnerable, and build a practice rooted in trust, impact, and empowerment. Touch becomes a declaration: "You are safe here. You are seen. You are supported."

CHAPTER 5

Boundaries and Balance in Massage Therapy

Touch is intimate. In massage therapy, it's a powerful tool for healing—but only when used within clear and ethical boundaries. Boundaries are not restrictions; they are containers for trust, safety, and professionalism. Balance, on the other hand, is the practitioner's ability to remain grounded and centered while holding space for others. Together, boundaries and balance make therapeutic touch both safe and effective. We have to think about the importance of boundaries and balance, not just in technique, but in mindset, energy, and practitioner-client dynamics.

Boundaries are the physical, emotional, energetic, and professional limits that define safe interaction. Boundaries can clarify what is appropriate and ethical, protect both the client and the practitioner, build trust and credibility, and leave a lasting impression on clients. In massage, boundary-setting begins before touch even occurs—through communication, intake forms, informed consent, and client education.

Types of Boundaries in Massage Therapy

- **Physical Boundaries:**
  - Respecting draping, positioning, and areas of the body that are and are not to be touched.

- o Never touching without consent.
- **Emotional Boundaries:**
  - o Recognizing when a client's emotional release is beyond the practitioner's role.
  - o Avoiding over-identifying or becoming overly involved in the client's emotional process.
  - o Maintaining awareness of your emotional energy and not absorbing the client's stress or pain.
  - o Practicing grounding techniques before and after sessions.
- **Time Boundaries:**
  - o Starting and ending sessions on time.
  - o Maintaining a healthy work-life balance and avoiding burnout.
- **Professional Boundaries:**
  - o Upholding ethical standards, confidentiality, and role clarity.
  - o Referring clients out when issues fall outside your scope of practice.

Boundaries communicate safety and build trust. When a client knows you will respect their limits, they are more likely to relax deeply, share their concerns and needs, return for future sessions, and refer your services to others. Without boundaries, trust breaks down, and therapeutic relationships become vulnerable to harm or miscommunication.

Regarding professional boundaries, massage therapist, Lidesyan "Dez" McKinney wasn't always sure how to establish them effectively. However, with experience as a long-term professional in the industry, she has clear rules, procedures, and policies in place, and firmly upholds her business principles, ethics, and goals. She ensures that all boundaries are now respected. Dez is a second-generation licensed massage therapist with over 15 years of experience. Her journey in the field began immediately after graduating from high school, a testament to her dedication and passion for her work. For Dez, building trust with her clients is not just a priority, but a commitment. As a Navy veteran and a trauma-informed therapist, she focuses on creating a comfortable and safe space for everyone she works with. Dez's dedication to understanding each client's unique needs and educating them on the potential benefits of massage therapy is a testament to how much she values her clients.

Balance is the practitioner's ability to stay centered—physically, emotionally, and energetically. It is essential because clients often bring heavy emotions and energy to the table. Practitioners must care for others without becoming depleted, and physical balance ensures safe body mechanics and longevity in practice. A balanced therapist communicates calmness and strength through touch. Clients can feel when a therapist is indifferent, distracted, tense, or overwhelmed. However, there are practices you can do to maintain balance by using grounding techniques, such as breathwork, visualization, meditation, or physical grounding exercises, before and after sessions. Then, you must think about your self-care rituals such as regular massage, movement, adequate rest, and nutrition. Time management is another component to avoid overscheduling and allow buffer time between clients.

Balance is not a one-time achievement—it's a daily practice. Clear communication is key to boundary-setting, and the best practices include explaining what to expect during the session, asking for consent before making adjustments, and encouraging clients to speak up if something doesn't feel right.

Phrases to use during appointments:

- "Let me know if the pressure is too much or too little."
- "Would it be okay if I place my hands here to help with your alignment?"

- "It's fine to ask for changes or breaks during the session."
- "Let me know if anything makes you feel uncomfortable, and it will be adjusted to your liking."

However, boundaries may be challenged when we encounter clients who are consistently tardy, request longer sessions without compensation, seek emotional support beyond our role, or exhibit inappropriate behavior. In such cases, stay grounded. You can respond with professionalism and clarity with the following statements.

- "I appreciate your openness, but this is outside my scope."
- "I can refer you to someone who specializes in that."
- "Our time today is set at 60 minutes. Let's make the most of it."
- "That behavior is not acceptable in this space. I'll have to end the session now."

If boundaries are still compromised, document any violations and seek support if needed. Effective practitioners walk a fine line between empathy and detachment. **Empathy** allows you to understand and connect with your client's experience, while **detachment** keeps you from becoming enmeshed or emotionally drained. Practicing compassionate presence means being fully with the client in the moment, while not carrying their pain after the session ends.

Shanese Armstrong, LMT, launched Well Kneaded LLC in 2013, and it was born out of her journey, with a solid team, serving over 1,000 individuals in Georgia. She builds trust with clients by being professional, consistent, approachable, flexible (to a point), a lifelong learner, and friendly. Armstrong established boundaries because she knows that first impressions matter, so it's essential to say what you mean and mean what you say, be consistent, be professional, and avoid letting things slip through the cracks. If something happens in the treatment room with a client overstepping boundaries, ensure you address it immediately, the first time, and redirect them. She knows that if you let things slip, they can get out of hand, and it's hard to regain control once it's lost. It's not impossible, just harder, so she trains clients and colleagues on how to behave, act, and respect you in and around the treatment room.

As a professional massage practitioner, you must not be afraid to say no because it is a powerful boundary tool. You're saying no to working beyond your capacity, no to requests that violate your ethics, no to performing modalities that you do not specialize in, and saying no to clients who drain your energy or disrespect your time. Saying no creates space to say yes to aligned, respectful, and fulfilling work.

Safe touch is empowering because boundaries and balance are not limitations—they are the framework that makes deep healing possible. They uphold client dignity and practitioner integrity, preventing burnout and emotional exhaustion. Lastly, as a practitioner, you're ensuring that every touch is given and received in safety, presence, and respect.

When boundaries and balance are honored, massage therapy becomes more than bodywork—it becomes a sacred exchange. In the next chapter, we will explore how presence and intuition enhance the quality of touch and deepen connection.

CHAPTER 6

The First Touch Is Trust: Foundations of Safe, Healing Contact in Massage Therapy

Touch is the bridge to trust because when our hands are safe, clients will begin to open their hearts. Before treatment, our hands have an unspoken agreement with the client because wellness starts with our hands. Before any technique is applied, before pressure is assessed, and before the first muscle is addressed, the foundation of every massage session is trust. The very first touch a massage therapist offers—whether a warm handshake, a grounding palm, or simply placing the sheet during draping—communicates a message. That message can either say, "You're safe here," or "Be cautious."

In the healing arts, the first touch isn't just physical—it's relational. It sets the tone for everything that follows, and if it doesn't establish trust, no amount of technical skill will reach the deeper layers of a client's nervous system. The human body is wired to respond to touch. Safe, respectful touch has been shown to release oxytocin, the hormone associated with bonding, trust, and safety. At the same time, it can reduce cortisol, the body's primary stress hormone.

The first touch matters more than the quantity or intensity. A hurried, mechanical touch can raise tension. A grounded, present touch can calm the mind, soften the tissue, and open the door to transformation. In essence, when you touch someone for the first time, you're communicating:

"I'm here with you. You can trust me.
Your body is safe in this space."

First impressions shape client experience; research in psychology shows that people form strong impressions within seconds of meeting someone. That includes massage clients. Your energy, presence, eye contact, tone of voice, and initial gestures all shape their first sense of comfort through a handshake or greeting, the way you listen during intake, how you invite them onto the table, and verbal tone when explaining the session. Trust is earned not only with your hands but with your presence.

Skylar Royal-Johnson, a massage therapist since 2013, is committed to a long and fulfilling career in the healing arts. He knows that trust is essential in client relationships and strives to make clients feel valued while providing the best possible therapy through an educational approach. As a male massage therapist, he is careful to establish clear boundaries before sessions, ensuring his presence and energy are always respectful and appropriate, while his professional demeanor commands respect.

Clients can feel when your mind is distracted. If your touch is rushed, uneven, or lacks presence, their body remains guarded. The first grounding contact should always be intentional, still, and calm. Grounded presence is a form of energetic hygiene. When your energy is centered and your attention is entirely in the room, clients will respond physiologically with a sense of ease. Touch is a language that speaks directly to the nervous system, bypassing words. A client's body is constantly scanning for signals, such as:

- Is this touch safe?
- Is this practitioner attuned to me?

- Can I relax, or do I need to protect myself?
- Is the session meeting my needs?

When your first touch is transparent, respectful, and attuned, it activates the parasympathetic nervous system, shifting the client from stress (fight or flight) into healing mode (rest and digest). This is not about performing—it's about being present.

A trusting relationship starts with informed consent, which means asking permission before beginning, offering options for positioning, draping, or modalities, asking about contraindications, or empowering the client to speak up or stop the session at any time. The simple question, "Is it okay if I begin here?" before placing your hands on a client's back, shoulders, or feet can build immediate trust. It shows the client they are in charge of their own experience. Every client comes to the table with their history, beliefs, and boundaries around touch. Factors to consider include trauma history, cultural values, personal modesty, and religious beliefs.

To build trust with the first touch, always approach with humility. Ask instead of assuming, respect differences, and allow the client's story to shape the session. It's not just where or how you touch—it's why. Touch to heal feels different than touch applied mechanically. Clients sense when your touch carries respect, safety, and the 4 C's: care, concern, compassion, and curiosity. As a practitioner, I encourage you to set an internal intention before your hands meet the client's body. Whether it's "I intend to support this client's release" or "May my touch offer comfort and peace," that intention will guide your hands with greater sensitivity.

10 Steps to Establish Trust Through Massage With Clients:

- **Professionalism:** Maintain a professional demeanor and appearance to create a trustworthy atmosphere.

- **Clear Communication:** Communicate the massage process, discussing any concerns or preferences with the client beforehand.

- **Informed Consent:** Ensure the client understands and consents to the massage, emphasizing respect for their boundaries.

- **Confidentiality:** Assure the client that their privacy and personal information will be kept confidential.

- **Skill Demonstration:** Showcase your expertise through skillful massage techniques to build confidence in your abilities.

- **Empathy:** Display empathy and actively listen to the client's needs, making them feel heard and understood.

- **Consistent Pressure:** Maintain consistent pressure during the massage, adjusting based on client feedback to enhance comfort.

- **Professional Environment:** Create a clean and comfortable environment that promotes relaxation and trust.

- **Check-In:** Periodically check in with the client to ensure their comfort level and address any concerns they may have.

- **Post-Massage Care:** Provide post-massage guidance, such as hydration tips or stretching exercises, reinforcing your commitment to the client's well-being.

Touch becomes transformational when massage therapists often witness incredible moments of healing that begin with a trusting touch. For example, a client with fibromyalgia, always guarded, finally exhales deeply after your steady palm rests on their back. You may have a client who survived trauma and shares that your calm presence made them feel safe in their body for the first time in years. A high-stress executive begins crying quietly mid-session—not from pain, but from relief. These moments don't come from advanced techniques—they come from trust, built at the very beginning or from various treatments.

Trust is a gift, given freely by the client, and it must never be taken for granted. As a licensed massage therapist, it is your ethical responsibility to maintain professional boundaries, use touch only with consent and clarity, and stay educated in trauma-informed and culturally sensitive care.

The first touch is not just a moment—it is the start of an ongoing, sacred agreement between you and the person on your table. Honor it with your presence. Protect it with your ethics. Deepen it with your intention. Trust is earned through touch, and healing becomes possible, not just for the body, but for the spirit in massage therapy.

CHAPTER 7

Mastering the Art of Touch with an Effortless Flow

The art of massage therapy is not just a science of pressure points and anatomy—it is also a fluid, intuitive dance between practitioner and client. An effortless flow in your massage session can emerge from the harmony between boldness, integrity, and presence. "Effortless flow" is a term often used to describe that seemingly natural ability some therapists have to move with grace, intuition, and confidence during a session. But this flow is not magic—it's the product of practice, presence, and mastery of touch. Effortless flow doesn't mean the work is easy; it means that the client perceives it as seamless. Your hands move with intention, transitions are smooth, and your presence is fully grounded. The client feels safe, cared for, and understood, without a word being spoken.

Effortless flow is a state of being, not just a technique. It comes from a grounded awareness where your mind, body, and intention are aligned. Your effortless flow allows you to trust your intuition and training. The movements are connected and fluid and present with the client's breath, body language, and needs. Flow is often described in psychology as a "peak experience"—time slows down, and action and awareness merge. As a massage therapist, entering this flow state deepens your ability to read your client's body and respond in real time.

Embodied awareness is a key skill for creating flow. It means being deeply in tune with your own body and breath while simultaneously attuning to your client. To develop this, we must practice self-care by stretching, exercising, participating in harmonious and adventurous activities, being physically grounded, and getting massages. Then, let your breath guide your pace and rhythm, and before sessions, do a quick mental check-in with your posture and presence. When your awareness is embodied, your touch becomes more present and intentional, which naturally creates a smoother experience for the client.

Effortless flow is built on strong technical foundations. Key techniques that support seamless touch include blending our five basic strokes while doing deeper work without abrupt changes. We can maintain contact by having a mother hand and a working hand. In other words, the massage therapist will keep at least one hand on the client whenever possible. As a practitioner, you must work with rhythm by syncing your pressure and movements with the client's breath or natural cadence. These techniques give your sessions an unbroken, wave-like quality that clients often describe as "meditative" or "soothing," and not robotic and stoic.

While technique is critical, intuition is what turns skill into art in massage therapy. Intuitive touch involves listening beyond words—paying attention to muscle tension, skin temperature, and energy shifts You must trust the subtle cues—sometimes, the body "asks" for more attention in certain areas. You have to stay flexible, especially when you have longer sessions, by adjusting your plan based on what you feel under your hands. Developing intuitive touch takes time, but the more you practice, the more naturally it flows, and it will be second nature.

Massage practitioners also consider the energetic aspect of touch because maintaining energetic balance contributes to a client's experience of flow. To master this concept, begin sessions with intention-setting or grounding and visualize energy flowing through your hands and into the client. It is essential to clear your energy before and after sessions to prevent countertransference. An effortless flow in massage can also be an energetic exchange—one that promotes healing on a deeper level.

Even experienced therapists encounter blocks to flow. Common issues include mental distractions, fatigue, or poor body mechanics. Worrying about timing or outcomes can pull you out of presence, and physical strain interrupts smooth movement. Failing to adapt to the client's unique needs can make your session feel mechanical. Solutions include mindfulness practices, regular bodywork for yourself, reducing stress, and continuous education to keep your skills fresh.

Clients may not always understand the technicalities of what you're doing, but they feel it. When your work flows effortlessly, clients often report that they're deeply relaxed and safe and just have a sense of being fully seen and supported. This is what sets exceptional and great massages apart for clients. When your flow aligns with the client's needs, you elevate the session from good to unforgettable.

To master flow, treat it like a daily practice and make it an everyday regimen by performing mindfulness exercises to center yourself before sessions and stretches to support physical ease and body awareness. Flow is a muscle, and the more you use it, the more fluid it becomes in your practice. True mastery in massage therapy isn't about knowing everything—it's about showing up fully in the moment. Each session is an opportunity to refine your touch, deepen your presence, and serve with heart.

Effortless flow is not about perfection; it's about connection. It's about allowing your hands to speak the language of healing with ease, rhythm, and grace. Your flow is your fingerprint. And when it's infused with integrity and boldness, the art of touch becomes a healing experience clients will never forget.

CHAPTER 8

The Science and Spirituality of Healing Hands

T he concept of healing through touch is an ancient and universal practice found across cultures and spiritual traditions. Whether through therapeutic massage or the biblical laying on of hands, healing hands have long symbolized the integration of science and spirituality in promoting wellness. This book explores both the scientific foundations and spiritual significance of healing hands, aiming to bridge the gap between modern medicine and ancient wisdom. Touch is the first sense to develop in humans and remains one of the most powerful modes of communication and healing. Scientific studies show that touch activates the parasympathetic nervous system, which helps the body rest, digest, and heal. Mechanoreceptors in the skin send signals to the brain, reducing cortisol levels and increasing oxytocin, dopamine, and serotonin neurochemicals that promote feelings of relaxation, trust, and well-being.

Massage therapy is one of the most recognized forms of healing hands in the medical field. It improves circulation, facilitates lymphatic drainage, and aids muscle recovery. Numerous peer-reviewed studies have demonstrated its efficacy in reducing pain, anxiety, and depression. Therapeutic touch used in massage is now commonly integrated into physical therapy and rehabilitation programs, showing tangible results that support its scientific validity. Beyond the physical benefits, healing touch is also believed to influence the human energy field, or biofield. According to energy medicine, the body emits electromagnetic and subtle energy fields that can be sensed and modulated through touch. Practices like Reiki, Therapeutic Touch, and Pranic Healing are based on the idea that practitioners can channel universal energy to balance and restore the client's biofield, thus supporting physical and emotional healing.

Although mainstream science often views energy healing with skepticism, emerging research is beginning to explore its effects. Studies using electroencephalography (EEG), thermography, and biophoton emission suggest that changes in energy patterns occur during healing sessions. While these findings are preliminary, they open the door to further scientific inquiry into how intention and energy interact with biological systems. Scientific studies in psychoneuroimmunology highlight how intention and emotional states influence immune function and overall health. Practitioners of healing touch often emphasize the importance of being fully present and setting a positive intention during healing sessions. This mindfulness and compassionate presence may significantly amplify the healing process by fostering trust and emotional safety in the client.

Spiritual traditions worldwide recognize the sacred power of healing hands. In Christianity, the laying on of hands is used for blessings and healing. In Eastern traditions, the hands are seen as conduits for life force energy, such as Qi in Chinese medicine or Prana in Indian Ayurveda. These practices often involve prayer, and meditation that invoke divine or universal healing energy. Numerous case studies and testimonials illustrate the transformative effects of healing hands. Patients report relief from chronic pain, emotional trauma, and stress after receiving energy-based healing or therapeutic massage. These personal accounts, while anecdotal, contribute to a growing body of qualitative data supporting the integration of touch-based therapies into holistic healthcare models.

Integrative medicine is a growing field that seeks to combine conventional medical treatments with complementary approaches such as massage therapy and energy healing. Healthcare providers are increasingly recognizing the importance of treating the whole person—body, mind, and spirit. Training programs for nurses, therapists, and physicians now often include education on the benefits of healing touch and mindful presence. Healing hands represent a powerful convergence of science and spirituality. Whether through measurable physiological changes or the more subtle shifts in energy and consciousness, touch can heal on multiple levels. As research continues to explore the mechanisms behind these practices, it becomes increasingly clear that the union of compassionate touch, scientific understanding, and spiritual intention holds great promise for the future of holistic healthcare.

CHAPTER 9

Continue to Cultivate Mindful Touch with Massage

M indful touch is the practice of applying intentional, conscious awareness during physical interaction, particularly through massage. It goes beyond technique, focusing on presence, empathy, and the therapeutic relationship between practitioner and client. In massage therapy, cultivating mindful touch fosters more profound relaxation, enhances healing, and supports the client's emotional and physical well-being. Mindfulness is defined as non-judgmental, present-moment awareness. When applied to massage therapy, it means being fully engaged with each stroke, each breath, and each client's unique needs. Mindful practitioners listen with their hands, attuned to subtle changes in muscle tone, temperature, and energy. This presence creates a safe, nurturing environment for healing.

Clients who receive mindful massage report a range of benefits, including reduced anxiety, deeper muscle release, enhanced trust, and a feeling of being truly seen and cared for. Mindful touch has also been linked to improved sleep, lowered blood pressure, and an increase in "feel-good" hormones such as oxytocin and serotonin, contributing to a holistic sense of wellness.

For therapists, practicing mindfulness during massage reduces burnout, increases job satisfaction, and fosters a stronger therapeutic connection. Staying present prevents mental fatigue and enhances intuitive decision-making. Therapists often find that mindfulness helps them maintain emotional boundaries while still offering compassionate care. Mindful touch can be developed through breath awareness, grounding exercises, and body scans before sessions. Therapists can pause briefly between techniques to recenter and ensure they are attuned to the client's needs. Using slower, intentional strokes also fosters mindfulness. Journaling or reflective practice after sessions helps deepen awareness and growth.

Scientific studies show that mindfulness and intentional touch activate the brain's limbic system, which regulates emotion and memory. When a therapist applies touch with awareness and compassion, it can influence the client's nervous system by reducing cortisol levels and increasing parasympathetic activity, promoting deep rest and healing. Mindful touch has roots in many ancient healing traditions, from Ayurvedic massage in India to the practice of Tui Na in China. These traditions emphasize presence, energy flow, and the sacred nature of touch. Integrating this historical wisdom into modern massage enhances the depth and intention behind each session.

Massage education programs are increasingly incorporating mindfulness into their curricula. Students learn to observe their breath, maintain ergonomic posture with awareness, and connect empathetically with clients. These practices support both technical excellence and emotional intelligence, creating well-rounded, intuitive therapists. Encouraging clients to engage mindfully during their sessions enhances the therapeutic outcome. Therapists can invite clients to focus on their breath, sensations, or emotions as they arise. Educating clients about the benefits of mindful touch empowers them to take an active role in their healing journey.

Cultivating mindful touch is an ongoing journey for massage therapists. It requires practice, reflection, and a commitment to personal and professional growth. By continuing to deepen awareness and compassion in their work, therapists can offer transformative healing experiences that nurture both body and spirit. Mindful touch is not just a technique; it is a way of being that honors the sacred connection between healer and client.

Epilogue

Massage therapy is a healing arts profession that is a lifelong practice that allows us to cultivate our touch with knowledge, skill, awareness, and ethical studies through continuing education courses. When these elements are established, the flow is effortless, and we can have an intuitive connection with clients through our skilled and purposeful touch. Trust must be established before a single hand is placed on the body. Touch is the cell membrane in massage therapy, but trust is the nucleus. Without it, even the most skilled hands can feel invasive, disconnected, or ineffective. With trust, however, your touch becomes a conduit for healing, connection, peace, and safety. The touch is meaningful and transparent, fostering client trust and presenting emotional security. The human body responds biologically to safe, therapeutic touch. Studies have shown that intentional, non-threatening touch reduces cortisol (stress hormone, increases oxytocin (the "trust" or "bonding" hormone) Lowers hypertension and heart rate, and activates the parasympathetic nervous system (rest and digest). However, these benefits only occur when the nervous system feels safe due to the practitioner's tone and manner of touch.

Massage therapy is a profoundly intimate experience. You are entering someone's personal space, touching their skin, and often addressing long-held stress or trauma stored in the body. But before you begin the treatment, the first impression matters as soon as the client enters your treatment room. The majority of the time, you don't get a second chance to make a first impression.

Trust begins the moment the client walks through the door—or visits your website. From the first phone call to the first hello, your professionalism, tone, and communication set the stage. There are several ways you can build trust through touch, such as a warm and confident introduction, a clean, productive, efficient, and welcoming space, a complete and thorough intake process, and listening to clients without judgment or ridicule. When the client feels seen, heard, and welcomed, their body begins to relax—even before your hands start their work. Once you begin the work, the body reads everything. Clients can feel if your mind is wandering, unaware of their needs based on your body language, rushed or anxious, or if you're grounded. Therefore, I am reminding massage practitioners, including myself, that when your touch is rooted in care and attention, clients feel it deeply. Trust is not just a concept—it's earned.

Nonetheless, trust starts with **informed consent** because clients must understand what will happen during the session and feel empowered to say yes or no. Clients trust therapists who are consistent, clear, and respectful of boundaries. It shows that you are dependable and safe. Touch is interpreted differently across cultures, ages, and identities. A trusting massage therapist is sensitive to religious or cultural views on physical contact, gender dynamics, and personal comfort, mindful about the preferences for draping or positioning. Asking rather than assuming builds trust. Cultural humility allows you to adapt and serve each client with deeper respect.

A trusting touch also respects the client's boundaries by starting and ending sessions promptly, asking questions, avoiding contraindicated areas, be mindful about draping, have clear scope of practice (no diagnosing or counseling), empowering the client to speak up at any time, checking in about pressure and comfort, and applying ethical and professional conduct at all times even when clients' attitude is unacceptable.

Boundaries create trust, and it's a form of protection, especially with trauma-induced clients. Statistics reveal that **1 in 5 people** have experienced some form of physical or emotional trauma. Trauma-informed massage recognizes this and adjusts accordingly by avoiding surprise movements or unexpected pressure, using grounding techniques (such as placing both hands gently on the shoulders before starting), paying attention to their breathing, and watching for non-verbal cues like muscle tensing or shallow breathing. For trauma-induced clients, trust is fragile; therefore, you must be empathetic, present, gentle, and respectful.

However, you may follow the right protocol and be mindful about your touch, but unfortunately, your touch may not align with everyone, and that's okay. People have preferences, but when you're transparent with a client, it shows your integrity, and you set the tone for a respectful and therapeutic touch. Sometimes, despite best intentions, trust is shaken and uncertain. Perhaps a client felt uncomfortable and didn't speak up, or a boundary was unintentionally crossed.

On the other hand, when the trust is compromised, apologize sincerely when you made a mistake, ask how to improve their comfort going forward, stay humble, and be open to feedback or constructive criticism. After the session, the client may or may not reschedule with you, but you can give them the opportunity to be heard and respected even after a misstep. You take the necessary steps to repair the client's trust and offer alternatives to fulfill their wellness experience.

When trust is present in your practice, whether it's a suite, spa, clinic, or wellness center, clients will revisit and refer others to your establishment. On a personal note, your confidence as a practitioner grows because the sessions will be therapeutic for yourself and the client. Establishing trust is not just good ethics—it's essential for a truly therapeutic experience. As a massage practitioner, you are in a sacred position. With your hands, you can help people release pain, reconnect with themselves, and feel safe in their bodies again. But it all begins with trust—earned, felt, and honored—one session at a time.

Massage therapy is more than touch—it's a conversation between the hands and soul, where tension fades and the spirit establishes peace. Remember, touch without trust in massage is just a technique, but with trust, it's a transformative treatment.

About the Author

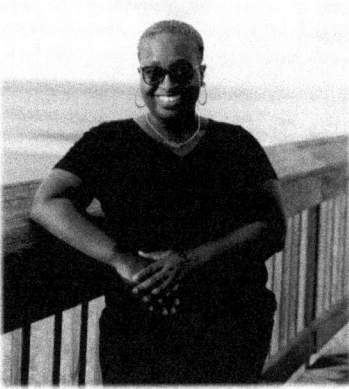

Dr. Dominique M. Carson, LMP, MMP, H.C is an award-winning and globally recognized freelance journalist, licensed massage practitioner, orator, and author. For over a decade, she interviewed over 100 notable figures in popular culture, such as Tito Jackson, Latto, H.E.R, Coco Jones, Jekalyn Carr, Jon B, Charlie Wilson, Regina Belle, Patti Labelle, Kirk Franklin, and many more. She also collaborated with Brooklyn historian and journalist Suzanne Spellen and launched a 118-page journal on Lefferts Manor, a neighborhood in Brooklyn. Carson also served as Program and Communications Coordinator for Man Up! Inc., a nonprofit organization in East New York, Brooklyn. While at the organization, she received a citation from the New York City Council and the "It's My Park Award" from the Partnership for Parks for community engagement in her hometown, East New York, Brooklyn. Her story has appeared in media outlets such as Sheen Magazine, Impact Magazine, Femi Magazine, Industry Times, and Forbes.One, VoyageLA, ShoutoutLA, and Bold Journey, to name a few. Carson's overall goal is to facilitate people's lives with her hands and words.

LinkedIn: https://www.linkedin.com/in/drdominiquemcarson/
Facebook: https://www.facebook.com/dmc922
Instagram: https://www.instagram.com/domcarson90
Website: Linktr.ee/dom0922

www.ingramcontent.com/pod-product-compliance
Lightning Source LLC
Chambersburg PA
CBHW071752050426
42335CB00065B/1782